EMERALD GUIDES

COMBATING CHILD OBESITY

OBESITY

Nicolette Heaton-Harris

Emerald Publishing
www.emeraldpublishing.co.uk

Emerald Publishing
Brighton BN2 4EG

Printed by GN Press Essex

9781847161239

Cover design by Bookworks Islington

Whilst every effort has been made to ensure that the information
contained within this book is correct at the time of going to press,
the author and publisher can take no responsibility for the errors or
omissions contained within.

Combating Child Obesity

CONTENTS

Introduction
Case Studies in Child Obesity

(All names have been changed for privacy and the opinions are not the authors or the publishers.)

"We'd taken Jodie to the doctor's because she was suffering from a viral infection and whilst we were there, the doctor had made this comment about her weight. It was only a little something. A bit offhand, about how she'd have an easier time breathing if it weren't't for the extra pounds she was carrying. At the time, I more concerned about her chest infection than anything else and it was only after, many weeks after actually, that his words came back to me.

I wasn't sure how Jodie would react to me taking away her sweets and crisps. She loved them so much and I liked giving them to her. I'd not had treats like that as a child. And I felt awful about restricting her. So I didn't I figured if I just took her to swimming lessons, that would be enough. They always say we all need to exercise more.

But it didn't work. The swimming made Jodie hungry and she'd want the chocolate from the machines when we came out. I know now, that if we want her to lose weight properly and healthily, then we have got to do both. Increase her activity *and* change her eating habits. It's going to be hard and quite frankly, I'm not looking forward to it. But I will, because it's for her own good."
(Harriet, 36)

"I'm always being picked last for things at school and I hate that! I like playing netball and doing gym, but no one wants to partner me or have me on their team. All the pretty girls get picked first. The thin ones. The ones the boys all like. I don't think any boys want to go out with me and why would they?

I'd love to lose weight. I really, really would. But it's so hard! I tell myself I can do it and I try not to eat that stuff. You know, chocolates and stuff. But it tastes so good! And it's hard doing it on my own. I don't tell anyone I'm doing it. I don't know why. I don't think they'will laugh, but I don't think they'd take me seriously. I think it would help if I had someone's support. Someone to keep an eye on me."
(Lyndsey, 15)

We've always given the kids big dinners. They're growing children, aren't they? They need it. It makes me feel good to put a big meal in front of them, because when I was little, we didn't get much. I spent most of my childhood feeling hungry!
(Sally, 30)

I hate being overweight. In the winter, you have to wear all these clothes to keep warm and I end up looking fatter than I am. But then, in the summer, when it's hot, I sweat like mad and I have to keep having showers and stuff. I get this really bad rash sometimes from the heat. It's itchy and prickly. I go all blotchy. I think I only really like autumn.
(Lyndsey, 15)

1

FACTS ABOUT OBESITY

Do you ever find yourself defending your child's weight? Whether to friends, family, or even in your own mind? Do you often find yourself saying/thinking, 'It's just puppy fat / They're big-boned / They'll grow out of it / They take after me'?

If so, then this book may be for you.

There have been a lot of reports in the media lately about childhood obesity and none of it is positive. The papers and news reporters repeatedly tell us that obesity in children is on the rise, that children are at risk of serious diseases if they do not lose their excess weight.

Well. Is it true? *Yes. It is.*

So it's all very well to tell us about a problem, to educate us about a problem, but what can we actually do about it, if we have a child that is overweight or obese?

This book will help you, as a parent, help your child in making informed choices about the food they eat, being active and have the motivation to keep going. Because losing weight is not easy.

Especially if you're used to being allowed to eat what you want, when you want. Especially if the child uses food to medicate themselves when they're feeling down or depressed.

But this isn't going to be a program just for your child. It's going to be for the whole family as a unit. And this is why:

FACT ONE : Many overweight children, have overweight parents

Let's look at this fact. It will not be true in *every single* case, but it seems to be true in the *majority* of cases. If a child, who is overweight, has overweight parents, then that child does not have good role models when it comes to food. Overweight parents will be eating too much of the wrong foods. Fatty, salty, calorie-laden foods. They may snack often, eat at the wrong times of day, drink lots of fizzy drinks or alcohol and serve huge portions because their child 'is a growing lad/girl'. These overweight parents will most probably be inactive. They won't exercise. They may order take-out and not eat fresh fruits or vegetables. Would it be any wonder their child is overweight too?

FACT TWO: Overweight/obese children usually become obese adults. Why? Well it only takes a moment to create a bad habit and sometimes years to break one. A child who has grown up in a home where they can eat unhealthy foods, have large portions, do no exercise and drink lots of pop and *do not have* informed parents who want to help their child, will continue to grow up through adolescence into adulthood without being able to change.

They get into a vicious cycle. By the time they've realized that they're overweight and their friends at school are making jokes and not wanting to pick them for a sports team, they know nothing better than to go home and make themselves feel better by eating chocolate or a packet of biscuits. They have no-one to motivate them to feel better about themselves or how to change, so this child grows up into an adult who either stays overweight and/or obese with massive health problems, or someone who yo-yo diets because they have no idea of self-control or support.

FACT THREE: Obese children are at risk of severe health problems

This is a scary one. Especially when you look at the list of what health problems can develop *just from carrying too much weight.* These problems are not there for any other reason. The problems develop because the child is overweight. That's it. Stark fact. If you do not help your child to change their eating habits and become more active, then your child will be at risk of developing one or more of the health problems I will go into in the next chapter. And let's not beat about the bush. Some of these problems can be fatal. And if you think I'm trying to scare you, then good. I probably need to scare you. I'm not over-dramatizing either. I just don't want Fact Four to happen.

FACT FOUR: Parents may soon start outliving their obese children

Just think about that for a moment. No one wants to outlive their children. Of course they don't. But if the problem of childhood obesity is not tackled, then this may very well happen. If you decide to ignore the 'puppy fat' and let your child grow up to become an obese adult, riddled with health problems and being at tremendous risk of heart failure, then you may very well end up burying your child.

FACT FIVE: Obese children are less active than the average pensioner

Can this be true? Yes, it can. Research by the BBC, revealed that the average child is less active in the average day, than an average pensioner. So let's think about that. We don't know exactly what the BBC classed as an average child, or an average day, or an average pensioner. But if you try to think about it, it's still pretty thought provoking.

Imagine a MR Smith, 70 years of age, touch of arthritis or angina. He gets up and ambles around his home getting ready to go out to collect his pension. He drives to the post office, perhaps, stands in line and talks to a few people. Then he goes shopping, pushing the trolley before going home to unpack. If the day is nice, he goes outside and does a spot of gardening, getting those weeds out of his rose bed or mowing the lawn. He might have a dog to walk or a game of bowls to go and play in the evening. Not incredibly active, but active all the same. He's not pounding away at the treadmill in the gym, but he is being active and that is something that the majority of overweight children are not. Okay, they may do P.E. at school, but do they put any effort into it? Do they try for about five minutes before they go all red in the face and huff and puff because they're out of breath? Do they run around and play at playtime?

Because MR Smith doesn't get out of breath after five minutes, but an overweight child will. Because of the strain on the heart to pump so hard around a too-large body that is demanding oxygen rich blood. Think about that.

FACT SIX: The average teenager eats three pre-packaged/ready meals per week

This includes takeaways and fast food too. Why is this? Why would a family need to pay for three (or more) takeaways or fast food per week? That's expensive. It would be so much cheaper to make their own pizza with fresh, healthy ingredients at home.

So why? It's because we live in an 'instant' culture. We expect, and demand, instant service. We have microwaves to cook food fast. We have drive throughs for those who can't be bothered to get out of their car and eat at a proper table. We have computers that instantly load games, when twenty years ago, you had to wait three or more minutes for your Spectrum to load up a tape cassette game. We have instant popcorn, frozen 'ready' meals, and tremendous amounts of instant gratification in this 'instant' society.

There is no patience. Think of road-rage. Think of stress levels. People today want stuff, and they want it now! They don't want to wait. Especially children. They ask and they are given. And this occurs with food. They don't have to wait for the ice-cream man to come round each tea-time, they can have a few tubs of it in the freezer and eat it at breakfast if they want to. They want some chips? They can microwave some in just a minute. They want a burger and fries? They can get one from the local take-away. In minutes, rather than wait for Mum or Dad to make some home made.

It's laziness. And impatience. But laziness is also a huge problem that contributes towards the even bigger problem of childhood obesity. The other problem with take-out food and ready-prepared meals are the high levels of salt. Too much sodium is also bad for the system, but eating a diet rich in salt can actually *alter* the taste sensations in your mouth. A body can get used to it and when you try to eat a food without salt, it can taste bland or awful to you, so you ignore it and keep with your salty requirements. Therefore buying more and more take-outs. Therefore ignoring the healthy salt-less foods.

These are just a few facts about obesity, but very important ones. I'm sure there are others, but I won't bombard you with information that you already know. Because you_*do* know that your child being overweight or obese in unhealthy. You do know that if you don't do something about it they're unlikely to change. And you also know that they're probably going to have health problems because of it. The first way to tackle a problem is to admit that there *is one*. And by picking up this book, then you've done that, otherwise you wouldn't be reading it.

So. There's a problem. You want to do something about it, but what? Perhaps you ought to know just exactly what you're up against?

What *might* happen if you fail to help your child?

Knowing the consequences of failure can be an incredibly motivating factor to actually succeed. So let's look at what problems can develop.

2

EFFECTS OF OBESITY

Being overweight or obese can cause many different types of health problems. Some of these can be incredibly serious. Dangerous. Even fatal. Some, say, varicose veins, may not seem all that terrible. They can always wear trousers, yes?

No. Why should they? Especially because you can start something now to prevent any or all of these problems from occurring because your child is overweight.

So, let's look at some of these health risks. I'll explain exactly what they are in simple terms and how each will affect the human body. What the short term and long term consequences are. What medications might be given to help with a problem and whether these have any long-term effects?

Because this is your child we may be talking about. And you don't ever like to think your child is in pain or suffering, do you?

Slipped Femoral Epiphysis
Sounds technical, I know. But basically, the femoral epiphysis is the ball of the hip joint in a child. The ball joint normally remains

positioned in the socket, however, if the join between the ball joint and the top part of the upper femur (thigh bone) weakens, it begins to slip and allows the affected leg to turn outwards, giving the effect of a bowed leg.

Overweight children between the ages of ten and sixteen seem to suffer from this more than any other and it also seems more prevalent in boys, than girls.

If a slip in the joint between the ball joint and femur occurs slowly (chronic condition) then the child is more likely to complain of pain in their groin area whenever they partake in exercise or some prolonged activity. They may even show signs of a limp, or have a slightly shortened leg. If that child then rests, the pain may gradually go away, or settle.

Some children may complain that their knees hurt with this condition and that is because the nerves that supply the hip, also supply the knee.

Occasionally, a sudden slip in the join, after a period of gradual weakening (acute condition) may cause severe pain in the child and cause difficulty in being able to walk. Thankfully, a sudden slip like this is rare.

In one case in three, both hips may be affected. But why do these slips (weakenings) occur? Well, they occur because the join between the ball joint and upper femur (growth plate) just cannot stand the stress that is placed upon it by obesity. The excess weight on such a joint, over a period of time, weakens the growth plate as it is not meant to take such weight or stress.

Treatment involves being admitted to hospital, where doctors will normally progress by starting with traction, using weights, but usually, surgery is required, a risk in itself upon an overweight person. During surgery, the epiphysis, is pinned. It can be a minor procedure, performed under general anesthetic, requiring a couple of small incisions in the upper thigh area, but if the slip is great and severe deformity of the joint and plate has occurred, the surgery can take longer and require a larger incision.

During the recovery period, your child would need crutches for about four to six weeks after the operation for mobility. They would be in hospital for about a week after the operation and after being discharged, would need to see specialists and have multiple X-rays whilst their bodies were still naturally growing. The long-term risk associated with slipped femoral epiphysis is that of degenerative arthritis in later life. Therefore, if your child complains of groin pain, limps, or complains about their knee or you have any concerns about them having this condition, the quicker you get them to see a doctor, the better.

Benign Intercranial Hypertension
Another technical sounding term. Fortunately, this is a very rare condition, but one that affects those who are overweight. The statistics on occurrence are about one in every two hundred

thousand, which isn't many, and doesn't sound too bad, unless of course, you're that one person who does have it, as the condition is not pleasant.

Benign Intercranial Hypertension (BIH) has two other names. Pseudotumour Cerebri (PTC) and Idiopathic Intercranial Hypertension (IIH).

This condition mostly affects women and its symptoms are many; headache, nausea, visual disturbances, memory problems, balance problems, tinnitus (a ringing noise in the ears) neck and back pain. The headaches from this condition can be continuous and in themselves, lead to irritation, mood swings, ruined sleep and depression

How is it diagnosed? With such a miss-mash of symptoms, you might not know you have a condition at all, so its worth being persistent when you see your doctor, especially since it is so rarely seen.

At a hospital, you will be given a CT scan or an MRI (magnetic resonance imaging) on the brain. The result for this scan will be normal, but might show signs of the ventricles in the brain being smaller than average. The next test is to measure the cerebrospinal fluid, by performing a lumbar puncture (a needle in the back). The results for this may show a raised level of fluid, though the protein, glucose and cell count may be normal. Next, there may be an examination of the eyes, which may or may not show a swelling of the optic nerve (papilloedema) with enlarged blind spots (though this last test may not show anything as sometimes with this condition the eyes may not be affected).

Treatment?

Weight loss. But what about whilst you're trying to lose weight? You may be prescribed Diamox, but as this can produce some very unwanted side effects (skin rash, skin peeling, itching, headaches, thirst, loss of appetite, pins and needles, mood changes, fatigue, dizziness, flushing and taste changes) you may be prescribed the different drug, Lasix.

The testing of the eyes (whether affected or not) is very important, as with this condition, blindness can occur if left untreated or undiagnosed and resulting surgery may be required.

After treatment and weight loss, prognosis is very good, although a few cases may be chronic and keep recurring, needing long-term medication and regular lumbar punctures to drain the high levels of cerebrospinal fluid.

Obesity Hypoventilation Syndrome

Obesity Hypoventilation Syndrome (OHS) is also called Pickwickian Syndrome and it occurs when an obese person does not breathe enough proper oxygen whilst they are asleep. Whereas you may think this sounds like sleep apnoea, it is a *form* of sleep apnoea (apnoea occurs to a person who may be overweight or not, causing them to stop breathing for a second or two, before suddenly starting again. This stop/starting may wake them).

OHS is caused because of a fault in the brain's control over breathing and an excessive weight against the chest wall, making it difficult for a sufferer to take a good lungful of air. Because they cannot take a deep breath, the blood loses oxygen and becomes over-rich in carbon dioxide which causes respiratory acidosis.

Patients with OHS will suffer from chronic fatigue caused by broken sleep, their sleep quality will be poor and some may develop chronic hypoxia (a bluish discolouration to the skin). Other symptoms may be excessive tiredness during the day, falling asleep in appropriate places such as work/school, having an increased risk of accidents because of a slow reaction response and depression.

Physical signs of OHS can be cyanosis (a bluish dicolouration to the skin, lips and nails) and right sided heart failure (which may or may not include swollen legs or feet, shortness of breath and fatigue after exertion).

If you suspect that someone has OHS, they can be tested through a sleeping study where they are monitored through a typical night and their pulmonary function and arterial blood gas is measured. Treatment is simply weight loss, but if this is not achieved, then mechanical ventilation can be used to help a sufferer breathe. This involves a mask that fits over the nose and mouth, forcing air into the airways. Or, more drastically, a tracheotomy may be performed. This is a small incision in the base of the throat, fitted with a device that keeps the hole open directly into the airway, though these can be troublesome and sometimes require suction.

If weight loss is achieved, then prognosis is good. If weight loss is not achieved and the patient continues to suffer with breathing, it can lead to serious heart problems, blood vessel complications, disability or even death.

Snoring

Snoring can affect anyone, man, woman or child, especially if they are overweight or obese. Snoring is caused by the soft palate at the back of the roof of the mouth vibrating because the air is not passing through the passages smoothly. During sleep, a person's muscles are relaxed and if they also have extra weight around their neck (which is usually the case in men who store fat here) then these tissues can sag under the weight, which stops the air flowing smoothly through. (Age can also be a factor with snoring. The older you are, the more likely you are to snore because your muscles have grown weaker over time.) Snoring can be treated through consuming a healthy diet and losing weight, performing regular exercise, sleeping on one side, not smoking and keeping the nasal passages open and clear. Complications can be many and also serious. For a start there is the effect that snoring has on others. Continually having to listen to someone snore, breaking *your* sleep patterns can cause friction and arguments. Marriages have been broken up because of a partner's snores. Then there are the medical causes; obstructive sleep apnoea, which in the long term can cause high blood pressure, strokes and heart attacks.

Snoring isn't so funny now, is it?

Varicose veins

Unsightly varicose veins mainly appear behind skin on the legs and are caused by veins that have twisted and swollen with blood. Thankfully for most, varicose veins are usually just a cosmetic problem that they either leave alone or have reduced by surgery or laser techniques, but for some unfortunate few, they can also cause some medical, physical problems. So how do they form?

All blood in the body is pumped around it by the heart and for the blood to be re-oxygenated, it must return to the heart. This means it has to flow upwards in the legs, fighting against the force of gravity. To ensure the success of this, the veins contain valves that point upwards, preventing blood from flowing backwards and these valves are aided by the leg muscles. Every time a muscle moves, it squeezes the deep leg veins, ensuring the valves push the blood back up the legs.

If blood does not flow correctly, it can pool and cause pressure in the thinner, surface veins and therefore you get the visible signs of varicose veins.

Being obese causes damage to the valves, though some people can inherit a trait that predisposes them to weak valves.

Symptoms include general aching and discomfort of the legs and sometimes, swollen ankles. Complications to develop from varicose veins is *thrombophlebitis*, where the veins become painful and reddened. They inflame and sometimes block the vein, though do not confuse this with Deep Vein Thrombosis (DVT), which requires hospital treatment.

Because of the nature of varicose veins, you must take care not to bump them or cut them as they can bleed profusely. If this occurs, you should apply basic first aid. Elevate the leg above the heart, apply pressure to the wound and call for medical assistance.

If you have great difficulties with varicose veins, a doctor can test the blood flow of the leg with ultrasound scans or issue you with compression stockings to be worn during the day. There is also a treatment called *sclerotherapy*, where the varicose veins are injected with a chemical that damages the vein walls, causing stronger leg veins to take over the blood flow, causing the damaged vein to reduce. Therefore it becomes less visible.

You could also consider surgery to remove the varicose veins under a general anaesthetic (bearing in mind the dangers of an obese person having an anaesthetic) or have laser treatment, which a lot of people report as being successful. However, none of this will be much use if your weight does not change.

Complications of varicose veins? Some people may develop painful, ugly leg ulcers and this tends to occur mainly in those who also have diabetes, another complication of being overweight. So to prevent varicose veins, you should avoid standing for too long, you should maintain regular exercise, wear compression stockings if varicose veins are already a big problem, but most of all, lose weight.

Gall bladder disease

The gall bladder lives on the underside of the liver and its general function is to store bile, which is used by the body to help with the digestion of fat.

GBD is unfortunately very common and mainly affects women. Symptoms are discomfort, severe pain after eating, jaundice, nausea and fever, and the most common reason for having GBD is the fact that you also have gallstones.

Gallstones are solid calcified stones formed in the gall bladder from cholesterol, bile fats and calcium. They can vary in size and form when the bile has too much cholesterol within it. With GBD and gallstones, you can suffer from three other uncomfortable conditions:

- Biliary Colic - this causes intermittent pains in the middle of the upper abdomen with the pain getting worse over an hour, before staying at the same, intense level. Pain then spreads to the right shoulder, between the shoulder blades and sometimes a sufferer can experience nausea, vomiting and excess wind. The biliary attacks can last from something as short as a few minutes, to a few hours and the attacks are frequent and severe. They are almost always triggered by eating fatty foods.

- Acute Inflammation of Gall Bladder - This is a persistent pain accompanied by a temperature that lasts for twelve hours or more. There is pain and tenderness under the right ribs and this pain gets worse with coughing, sneezing or any other trunk movements. It requires hospital admission and antibiotics to treat the inflammation or surgery to remove the gall bladder.
- Jaundice - With this, the body increasingly becomes yellow and the skin becomes itchy. The motions are pale and urine turns dark. It is sometimes accompanied by shaking, fever and chills.

So what to do? You can get over the counter painkillers to deal with mild attacks of pain or you can apply something warm to the abdomen. The main thing is to introduce a low-fat diet and eat healthily. A doctor will diagnose gallstones from a blood test that checks upon liver function. Then there are the ultrasound scans, CT scans (computerised tomography) and MRIs.

Treatment, as stated before, is a low fat diet, or eventually surgery, again with the risk of anaesthetic if you still remain overweight. There is also *dissolution therapy* (though stones must be small and of a certain type) where the stones are dissolved, *lithotripsy* (blasting small stones using a beam of sound and the remaining fragments removed through dissolution), or surgery.

Cholecystectomy is the name for removal of the gall bladder. If the gall bladder is kept after therapies or treatments, there is a high chance of stones reoccurring.

Polycistic Ovarian Syndrome

If you are diagnosed with PCOS, then know that it is treatable, if not curable. It is mainly treated through medication and a change in diet and exercise. Symptoms are quite well known, irregular or absent periods, ovarian cysts, high blood pressure, acne, elevated insulin levels, diabetes, infertility, excess hair yet thinning of scalp hair (alopecia), skin tags and sleep apnoea.

PCOS can be diagnosed through many different tests. A doctor will complete a full health history, give a pelvic exam, perhaps do an ultrasound and test the blood. Birth control pills can help regulate hormones and try and control weight and excess hair. If you are diabetic as well, then your diabetes medication may also help with this. There are medications to help reduce hair growth and if you try and reduce and maintain a healthy weight, your bodies glucose levels will drop and your insulin will be used more effectively by the body systems. Periods will also be restored. Even a loss of 10% of body weight can help regulate a woman's monthly cycle.

Complications of PCOS include a higher risk of some cancers, diabetes, high cholesterol, high blood pressure and heart disease. If you're still overweight and suffering after the menopause, symptoms may get worse.

High blood pressure

Most people know the importance of maintaining a healthy blood pressure. Blood pressure is simply the measure of pressure of blood in your arteries. 140/90mmHg is considered high, but it has to routinely be this high after being tested many times before you are diagnosed as having high blood pressure. If it is 160/100mmHg or above, then you are considered as having very high blood pressure and you will be prescribed medication to control it. If you are given blood pressure medication, you will be on it for life and have a significantly higher risk of cardiovascular (heart) disease, diabetes and organ damage.

The pressure will depend upon how hard the heart has to pump and how much resistance is in the arteries. If the arteries are narrowed, then there is resistance to the blood flow, which then increases the blood flow. If you are overweight, eat a lot of salt, ignore fruit and vegetables and don't exercise, then you are at tremendous risk of high blood pressure. And you won't know you have it, unless you are tested for it. HBP is a recognized cause of cardiovascular disease, kidney damage, artery damage and heart strain.

If you want to try and lower your BP, you should lose weight, eat healthily (including at least five portions of fruit and vegetables daily), cut out salt and see if your doctor thinks you need medication. Even on medication and after weight loss and a healthier diet, you will have to have regular blood pressure checks.

High cholesterol

High cholesterol is called h*ypercholesterolaemia.*

Cholesterol is one of our bodies fats, also called lipids, and cholesterol is actually an important building block of the body (despite all our worries about it) containing triglyceride in the structure of the cells, as well as being important in making hormones and producing energy. This is why there are both 'good' and 'bad' cholesterols.

To some extent, your cholesterol level can depend upon what you eat, but there are other reasons too, such as how the individual body makes cholesterol in the liver. Having too much bad cholesterol in the blood is not a disease in itself. But it leads to other problems such as hardening and narrowing of arteries (atherosclerosis).

So what are the differences? Good cholesterol is known as HDL (high density lipoprotein) and the bad cholesterol, which is a large problem for those overweight or obese, is called LDL (low density lipoproteins). HDL has a useful job in the body by reducing the cholesterol in the tissues and taking it back to the liver and therefore protecting against the atherosclerosis, whereas LDL may contribute towards a person developing cardiovascular (heart) disease.

It is the *proportion* of LDL to HDL that influences the degree to which a person may develop a problem with their health. But fortunately, LDL can be lowered and controlled by eating a low fat diet and if needed, taking medication. Another good point to note, is that the good cholesterol, HDL, can be raised through exercising.

So how do doctors measure a cholesterol level? What do they consider 'high'?

- Less than 5mmol/L   =   an ideal level
- Between 5 to 6.4mmol/L   =   mildly high level
- Between 6.5 to 7.8mmol/L   =   moderately high level
- Above 7.8mmol/L   =   a very high level

Doctors will take a sample of your blood and send it off for testing. Results may take a day or two to come through, though there are home testing kits available from pharmacies that vary in price. Things to be taken into consideration are the facts that cholesterol levels can naturally rise with age, or be high within certain families or even influenced by the area in which you live! Geographically, Northern Europe has higher cholesterol levels than Southern Europe and Asia. This points some way to the way that different people cook and prepare foods. The relationship to food can be important, but your genetics and health history will play some part in what level you have and all of this will be taken into consideration by your GP.

So what can you do if you have a high cholesterol level?

You can change your diet, not smoke, reduce alcohol intake, exercise more, maintain a healthy diet and lifestyle and avoid being overweight.

Statins can be prescribed by your doctor as a medication, but some of these have side effects, such as muscle pain and bloating and if you do have any problems then you need to go back to your doctor.

Type2 diabetes

Another name for this is *diabetes mellitus*, or 'sugar diabetes'. Essentially, it is a long-term condition caused by the body's inability to regulate the amount of glucose present in the blood and it no longer reacts to the hormone insulin or notices when insulin levels are too low. Strangely, Type 2 diabetes is a condition that you can have and not know it. It often shows no symptoms at all and tends to be picked up by other blood tests. Though occasionally, when a sufferer has had the diabetes for a long time without being controlled, it can lead to signs of excessive thirst, the need to pass urine more frequently and weight loss.

Fortunately, Type 2 can be controlled with diet, exercise or medication, but if it is poorly managed it can lead to a greater risk of heart disease, stroke, nerve damage and even blindness. Glucose is absorbed from food and drink and is also produced in the liver. When the glucose in the blood reaches the tissues of the body, it is converted to energy. This concentration of glucose level, is managed by insulin, the hormone secreted into the blood by the pancreas. When there is a shortage of insulin, the glucose builds up and up in the blood, leading to the symptoms of diabetes.

If you are over 40 years of age, or are very overweight (especially as a child) then you are at risk of Type 2 diabetes. Being overweight, means a BMI (body mass index) of 25 and having a sedentary lifestyle. Type 2 can also run in families so genetics plays a part. And if you have a high blood pressure and/or high cholesterol too, then you run an even greater risk of developing Type 2 diabetes.

Be aware that two thirds of people with Type 2 will show *no symptoms*. But there are signs to look for such as the need to urinate, being excessively thirsty, losing weight, having an increased appetite, feeling sick and nauseous, having blurred vision and developing infections such as thrush.

Type 2 can be diagnosed from your doctor taking a full medical history, including that of close relatives, a physical examination, a blood test to measure glucose or asking a patient to take part in a glucose tolerance test.

Thankfully, it is a condition which can be treated, once diagnosed. You need to change your lifestyle and start on a healthy diet which includes one low in saturated fats, low in sugar and salt, but high in fibre, vegetables and fruit. You will also need to exercise, maybe take medication or have insulin injections. Your blood glucose levels will be monitored often, but most importantly, you will have to keep your weight under control.

Heart failure

Heart failure is initially caused by coronary artery disease (CAD) and hypertension.

Atherosclerosis (the hardening/narrowing of arteries caused by high cholesterol) is the main cause of coronary artery disease. A partial blockage of a main artery would cause angina and chest pain or pressure. This is caused by a weak, inadequate delivery of oxygen to the heart tissue. The plaque increases the risk of blood clots forming and a total blockage of an artery would cause a myocardial infarction (heart attack).

CAD is not just a problem caused by a diet, but it is a major factor. CAD can also be linked to genetics and age, but your lifestyle and general health, if unhealthy, can start the process of its development a lot more quickly, especially if you smoke, don't exercise, eat badly and also have other conditions such as diabetes or high cholesterol.

So what are the symptoms?

Swollen legs and ankles, shortness of breath (especially if you are laying flat), angina and general fatigue.

So how is it treated?

Angioplasty is usually the first treatment, but there is also bypass surgery and significantly, lifestyle change.

Heart failure can be worsened due to poor diet and lifestyle and factors that contribute greatly to heart failure are; family history, diabetes, obesity, heavy alcohol use, failure to take medication, large salt intake, large fat intake and sustained rapid heart rhythms.

It can be diagnosed through a chest X-ray, echocardiogram, electrocardiogram, tracer studies, treadmill test and catheterisation.

Coronary heart disease

CAD occurs when the arteries that supply blood to the heart muscle become clogged, hardened and narrowed with plaque that slowly builds up upon the inner walls. This build up is known as atherosclerosis. When this occurs, the blood flow to the heart is vastly reduced and can result in the patient experiencing angina pains or even heart attack. As time passes, the weakened heart becomes vulnerable to possible heart failure and a vast range of arrhythmias (changes in beat) which can be quite serious in themselves.

The atherosclerosis is caused by the plaque and the plaque is made up from excessive amounts of fats, cholesterol, calcium and other substances found in the blood. This build-up can begin in childhood.

There are two types of plaque, hard and soft. Hard plaque attaches itself to the walls of the arteries, causing them to harden and thicken, reducing blood flow and raising blood pressure. This type is associated with a sufferer becoming a casualty of angina and possible heart attack. The soft plaque is just as dangerous and unstable. It can break off in pieces from the interior walls of the arteries, leading to clots and eventual heart attack.

Those at risk are those mainly over 45 years of age and if there is a family history of heart disease or problems, having a high blood pressure, high blood cholesterol, if you smoke, have diabetes, are overweight or obese and do not have an active lifestyle.

The most common signs and symptoms of CAD is chest pain and discomfort, angina, pain in one or both of the arms, especially the left arm, left shoulder, neck and jaw, back pain with shortness of breath.

Unfortunately, sometimes, the only sign, and first sign, of CAD is a heart attack.

If you suspect CAD, then it can be diagnosed through various methods. Electrocardiogram, echocardiogram, stress tests, chest X-ray, cardiac catheterisation, coronary angiography and a nuclear heart scan. But to prevent CAD, the best things to do are be aware of your family health history, maintain a healthy weight and lifestyle, eat well and exercise.

Heart attack

This will occur when the supply of blood and oxygen to an area of heart muscle is compromised or blocked, usually by a clot somewhere in the artery. This blockage can lead to arrhythmias first, that cause a severe decrease in the ability of the heart to pump effectively. This can even lead to sudden death. If the blockage is not suspected and treated within hours, then the affected heart muscle will die and be replaced by scar tissue.

Warning signs of a heart attack, include, chest discomfort, jaw and neck pain, shortness of breath, cold sweats, nausea and vomiting, light-headedness and dizziness. Sometimes there may be no signs.

Heart attack is usually brought on by atherosclerosis, taking cocaine, stress, cold exposure and smoking. If you are over 45 years of age (men) or 55 years of age (women) and have a family history of heart problems, personal history of angina, have had a previous heart attack, or a surgical procedure like a cardiac angioplasty or bypass, then you are at greater risk of an heart attack. The risk factors you can change to reduce your risk, are, stop smoking, reduce blood pressure, reduce blood cholesterol levels, lose weight, become more physically active and be aware if you have Type 2 diabetes.

Therefore, the best way to prevent heart attack is to eat healthily, maintain the correct weight for your height and build, and if you have had a previous heart attack, ensure you make the correct lifestyle changes (diet, exercise, lose weight).

Osteoarthritis

Osteoarthritis is the most common joint disorder that is located in the hands, knees, hips, back and neck. It is caused by the breakdown of cartilage between the joints, a problem which is usually hastened by the added stress placed upon the joints from extra weight and stress.

The implications are clear. Being overweight hastens the breakdown of cartilage and once the joints have suffered this kind of damage, there will always be problems with those joints. The only way to help manage the pain and discomfort, apart from taking medication when needed, is to lose weight to lessen the problem of the lode-bearing stress.

Chafing

Skin chafing can happen suddenly, or it can become worse over a longer period of time. A sufferer can become aware of it through experiencing a sudden, stinging or burning sensation, caused by two areas of skin, rubbing together constantly. The inflamed surfaces of skin can actually, over time, be rubbed away and become raw, leaving a person with open wounds, skin sores, ulcers and ultimately, bad infections. Chafed skin needs time to heal and dry out. There are powders and medications for mild cases that can treat the irritated skin and special, stronger medications if fungal infections have set in to the worn area. Chafing can be prevented through wearing looser clothing, sweating less, using medication, but most effectively by losing weight.

Sweating

Sweating excessively is called *hyperhidrosis*. Normal sweating is essential for anyone. It helps to aim body temperature control, but for some people, it can become an uncomfortable and unsociable condition. Excessive sweating can lead to skin chafing and poor body odour and infection setting in, but it can be treated and/or masked with anti-perspirants and deodorants. But essentially, maintaining a healthy weight, so that the body does have to go into overdrive to cool an overly large body, would help this problem immensely.

Anesthetic risks

Having an anesthetic is a risk for anyone, but it is even more so if you have an excess of weight or are obese.

An anesthetic works by blocking the signals of pain or sensation that are normally sent along the nerve pathways and in the case of a general anesthetic, you are also asleep.

If you are overweight and know you are going to have an anesthetic, you should try to lose weight before the procedure and actually, some surgeons may *refuse* to operate on you until you do so, because of the higher risk of your heart stopping under anesthesia. This occurs because when you are lying flat and have so much excess weight laying flat against the chest wall and abdomen, it adds complications towards getting adequate airflow into your sedated system.

Stretch marks

These skin marks are caused by thin, stretched tissue and usually occurs in those that gain weight fast or lose weight fast. The upper layer if a person's skin is normal, but the lower layers of collagen and elastin become thin and stretched, then broken. Firstly, the marks are bright red or purple and can appear quite vivid to the eye, but after time, these marks fade to a silver-white which is simply the fat under the skin showing through.

Try to avoid yo-yo dieting which makes the problem worse. Stretch marks are permanent.

Asthma

Asthma is a condition that affects a person's airways. It is caused by a trigger, individual to that person, that irritates the airways, tightening the muscles so that they narrow and inflaming the passages so that they swell. Sometimes there can even be an excess of mucus or phlegm production too.

Asthma symptoms are common. Coughing, wheezing, being short of breath and having a tightness across the chest.

There is no cure for asthma and so if you are diagnosed and given medication, you must ensure you use it properly and effectively. There are different kinds of inhalers and depending upon the type of asthma you have, you may be prescribed a variety of types to be used in different situations. (Reliever inhalers, preventer inhalers, steroid tablets, spacers and nebulisers.)

There are hardly any side effects to asthma medication and generally they are very safe to use. Some of the relievers can temporarily increase your heartbeat or give you mild muscle shaking and trembling and with the prevention inhalers there can sometimes be a small risk of a sore tongue, throat, a hoarseness of voice or even oral thrush.

If you are given the steroid tablets you should be made aware that long term use can lead to a lower resistance to the chicken pox virus, give you mood swings and increase your hunger. You can also sometimes feel hyped up or depressed, have a fattened (moon) face, have difficulty sleeping, experience heartburn, indigestion, bruise more easily, alter any diabetic control medication, give you a risk of cataracts or brittle bones.

The ways in which you can manage asthma for yourself are to get fit, lose weight, exercise regularly, take your medication properly, stop smoking and cut down on unnecessary stress.

SUMMARY

It is quite clear that so many of these problems could be helped (or even avoided) by not being overweight or obese. Many of the conditions can start in childhood, but not show any symptoms until adulthood and a lot of the conditions are interconnected. If you have one, you seem more likely to also have another. And this can all be down to weight and lifestyle.

This is crucial. And very important to remember. Some of these conditions may seem minor, like chafing skin, or excess sweating. But a lot of these conditions can be a great risk to the health or even kill you. And it could all be altered by what passes your mouth and how you live your life.

But not all people who are overweight or obese are like this because they eat too much or don't exercise. Some people have medical conditions that cause them to be overweight and we'll explore them next.

3

MEDICAL CONDITIONS THAT CAUSE OBESITY

Not everyone who is overweight is like that because they enjoy fat-laden food and eat too much. There actually are medical conditions that can cause some people to be overweight and if that is the case, then this chapter is for you.

But even if you do have a medical condition that predisposes you to being overweight, that doesn't mean that you can just accept that and say 'oh, I have a medical condition. It's not my fault.' Because you can still manage that condition and do what you can to help with the weight problem. Just because you have, say, Prader-Willi Syndrome and that is the cause of you being overweight, it does not mean that you will not suffer from the problems mentioned in the previous chapter. You will be at just as much as a risk as those without a medical condition to start with! So, let's explore those conditions, see what causes them and acknowledge them, and then we'll get on with what you can do to help yourselves.

Prader-Willi Syndrome
This syndrome is a complex genetic disorder that is present from

birth. The main characteristics found in people with PWS are an excessive appetite, low muscle tone, emotional instability, immature physical development and learning disabilities.

The intense interest in food seems to become noticed in the first four years of life. Children have an insatiable appetite, eating everything and anything and will do whatever they can to obtain food, without worrying about consequences.

This need can be managed though, through good dietary control and educating the child, though lapses may still occur. Weight gain is rapid for someone with PWS and if calorie intake is not controlled, fat can accumulate quickly on their bodies as they have less need for calories than other people. By the time PWS sufferers become teenagers, their weight problems are usually obvious and sometimes, life-expectancy can be low if the PWS is not controlled efficiently, but there have been many sufferers who have lived past middle age.

The excessive appetite is known as h*yperphagia* and it is caused by a hypothalmic dysfunction. The messages that a person had eaten enough does not get through to the brain and so the person constantly feels hungry.

Appetite suppressants have been shown to have little effect on PWS sufferers and so diet management seems to be the best way to control this syndrome before other obesity-related diseases cause problems.

Hypothyroidism

This is caused when the body lacks enough of the thyroid hormone. The condition where people say 'I have a problem with my glands'.

The thyroid's main job is to regulate the body's metabolism and when this is thrown into disarray, then problems occur.

Hypothyroidism can be caused by inflammation of the thyroid gland. This inflammation damages or even destroys the cells within the gland leaving them dead. A person's own immune system can also cause damage to the thyroid (autoimmune thyroiditis) and also medical treatments wherein part or all of the thyroid is removed, can affect the system.

Symptoms of hypothyroidism are fatigue, weakness, weight gain, dry hair, pale skin, dry skin, hair loss, an intolerance to the cold, cramps, constipation, depression, irritability, memory loss, abnormal menstrual cycles and a decreased libido. Though some patients may have no symptoms at all. But this is a condition that requires a doctor's supervision. The body expects a certain amount of thyroid hormone, so if it not working properly, the pituitary gland will make an excess of TSH (thyroid stimulating hormone) to up the production. Constant high levels of TSH can enlarge the gland and form a goiter. If untreated, the symptoms of hypothyroidism will increase. This condition is rarely life threatening, but had been known to cause heart failure and coma.

It can be diagnosed through a simple blood test and treated with medication.

Cushing's Syndrome

This is a hormonal disorder, caused by prolonged exposure of the body's tissues to high levels of cortisol.

It *is* rare, but many people are still diagnosed with it each year.

Symptoms vary, but include; upper body obesity, a rounded face, increased fat around the neck and thin arms and legs. Children with this condition tend to be obese with slow growth rates and their skin becomes very fragile. They bruise easily and heal badly. Stretch marks form easily and bones weaken, giving aches, pains and are prone to fractures. There can also be severe fatigue, weak muscles, high blood pressure, high blood sugar levels, irritability, anxiety and depression.

The cortisol's role in our body is to help maintain our blood pressure and our cardiovascular functions. It also reduces our immune system's inflammatory response, balances the effect of insulin in the body, regulates the metabolism of proteins, carbohydrates and fats and also helps our body when responding to stress.

Most cases of Cushing's Syndrome are caused by pituitary adenomas. These are benign tumors located in the pituitary. Also, an abnormality of the adrenal gland can cause Cushing's. In the main, it is not usually an inherited condition.

It can be diagnosed through a medical history, a physical examination, laboratory tests, X-ray and a 24 hour collection of urine to test for cortisol levels.

Treatment may involve surgery, radiation therapy, chemotherapy or cortisol inhibiting drugs, depending on your type of Cushing's.

Syndrome X

This is a nutritional disease caused by eating the wrong types of food and the body's inability to deal with the types of food eaten. If you have Syndrome X, you may have symptoms that cause you to age prematurely, be obese, suffer with hypertension, have disorders of the nervous system, eye problems, diabetes, cardiovascular disease, cancer or even Alzheimers.

You may feel exhausted for most of the time, disorientated and depressed, irritable and have mood swings. Your body may become insulin resistant and you may develop Type 2 diabetes.

The main treatment for Syndrome X, is to control your diet and exercise.

Frohlich Syndrome

This is an extremely rare childhood metabolic disorder that causes obesity, growth retardation and under development of the genitals. It is primarily caused by tumors in the hypothalamus which in turn cause an increased appetite and a decreased secretion of gonadotrophin.

Bardet Beidl Syndrome

This condition is usually diagnosed during childhood after significant eye problems are experienced. The first symptom is usually a night blindness, followed by a loss of the peripheral vision. But another vital piece of information which will point to Bardet-Biedl, is the fact that the child was often born with extra fingers or toes, as well as being an overweight baby.

The obesity present in childhood leads to an increased risk of kidney disease. This condition can be passed down through family members.

Treatments for the eye problems are carried out on an individual basis, depending on the severity experienced.

Borjesson-Forssman-Lehman Syndrome

This is also a rare condition that apart from obesity, causes severe intellectual disability, epilepsy, coarse facial features, long, elongated ears and a shortness in height. Babies are born obese and very floppy and during childhood, the sufferers usually experience problems in school. Treatment is usually testosterone supplements.

Cohen Syndrome

This is also known as Pepper Syndrome. The major factors of suspicion for Cohen Syndrome are obesity, delayed mental development and delicate hands and feet. A small number of patients with Cohen's have heart defects, mainly affecting the mitral valve and their puberty is somewhat delayed. (Obesity does not always occur in every case of Cohen's.)

Insulinoma

This is a difficult condition to diagnose. It is caused by a tumour that produces excessive amounts of insulin. Almost all of these tumours are benign.

Symptoms can include blurred vision, palpitations, confusion and disorientation, amnesia, sweating, hunger or unconsciousness. The symptoms of an insulinoma can be aggravated by someone consuming a high-calorie diet, but the condition can be treated, usually through surgery and medications.

Melancortin 4 Receptor Defect

This defect affects the body's ability to efficiently store and use energy and therefore causes extreme obesity.

Pseudohypoparathyroidism Type 1A

With this condition, patients have a growth hormone deficiency and are therefore, typically short and obese. As you can see, there are many medical conditions, though often rare, that can be a contributing factor towards obesity.

However, just because your child may have been diagnosed, with say, Prader-Willi, or any of the others, this does not mean that they are immune to the effects of obesity as described in Chapter Two. A parent cannot think that just because a disease or syndrome is causing the obesity, then their child will not suffer from cardiovascular problems or diabetes or any of the others. Where there is obesity, there is risk to health. And so with knowledge, motivation and determination to control the weight and health aspect of a child's life, a parent, child, or family group can work together to improve a child's prospects and longevity of life.

4

MOTIVATION AND SELF-ESTEEM

"My Dad had been trying to give up smoking after a doctor told him that his bad chests were caused by all the cigarettes he kept getting through. But every time he tried, he'd start smoking again after about a week. He said he couldn't help it. He tried everything. Patches, nicotine gum. But nothing worked. He said he felt like he was doing it all alone. Which he was. I needed to lose weight. So we helped each other to keep going. Everytime Dad wanted a smoke, he'd tell me and I'd occupy his mind with a word game or we'd go for a walk and everytime I wanted some chocolate or a snack, Dad would show me a magic trick or we'd have a game of kickabout in the back garden. We kept each other going and it was easier to do when we weren't doing it alone."
(Daniel*)

It takes seconds to create a bad habit and often weeks, months or even years to kick it, no matter what that bad habit may be. Whether smoking, drinking, or in this case, eating too much, snacking on calorie, fat-laden foods and being lazy. And the main problem with a bad habit, is that it is often one that you have created all by yourself and so to be rid of it, you also think you have to do it all by yourself. For a child that is overweight, used to snacking on chocolate, crisps or biscuits, asking them to kick that habit and start eating healthily and exercise a little self control as well as starting to become more active, is a mission impossible.

They do not have the motivation or the knowledge on how to do that by themselves. Especially if they are very young. They may think they can do it, and even be a little bit excited by the challenge, but as with most promises to the self (think of New Year Resolutions) we start off feeling confident about our ability to change something, but as time goes by and the novelty of such a venture wears off, we lapse in our behaviours and fall back into old ways.

And food provides such a comfort, doesn't it?

Think about it. A lot of parents react to an upset child by offering it a biscuit or a sweet to 'cheer them up' and take their minds off the fact that they were upset because they fell and scratched their knee or their sibling pushed them or called them a nasty name. A parent may offer a crying baby a nipple to suck on, or a bottle, in an effort to soothe the upset child. And quite often, the baby or child will quieten at this sudden, wonderful gift. This act, done so innocently and with the best of intentions, becomes rooted in memory.

If you are upset, eat something.

Can you see how easily it is done? And if this habit begins in babyhood, then just think of how long that bad habit has become ingrained in your child. They have no other idea of how to make themselves feel better. They may come to you for a hug, or a kiss and a cuddle, but they will also want food. And, as the parent, you give it to them, because you don't want your child to be upset.

So when a child goes to school and gets picked on or bullied for being overweight and unfit, that child does not have you there to provide comfort and so eats sweets, or crisps, or whatever food they have available to them. They self-medicate, without realizing that the very medicine they are giving themselves, is actually the thing making their situation worse!

Children cannot be expected to know about good foods at such an early age unless you have taught them.

If a child eats lots of sweets or consumes lots of sugary drinks, then it will be hard for them to change their eating habits because their taste buds will come to expect those sweet flavors and sensations from all foods. Anything plain, like an apple, say, may seem horrible to them because it just isn't sweet enough. Even though apples are naturally sweet, a child can become accustomed to the artificial sweetness that is in so many unhealthy foods. And let's remember, a child is not the one with the buying power. A child does not go to the supermarket and put the foods in the trolley and pay for it at the till. *You do.* You are the one with the buying power. You make the choice of what goes in the trolley and you are the one that has to be strong enough to say, *I'm not going to buy those types of unhealthy foods anymore.*

I'm not advocating you make your child go cold turkey. That would seem incredibly harsh and everyone is allowed a treat now and then. But if you normally buy a 12-pack of crisps to get your child through the week, just buy two single packets. Or even one. Eventually this one packet can be phased out too, but to start with, it helps the child to know that they aren't being punished and if you withdraw all of their 'treats' straight away, you will often end up with a very uncooperative child in your home.

Or does some of the problem lie with you? Do you feel the need to give your child huge portions of food because 'they're growing'? Are you feeding a need within yourself? Or are you letting your child have whatever they want to eat, including all those sweets and chocolates whenever they want, because it was something *you* never had as a child?

Food can become an addiction and it is up to the whole family to break it.

But how?

Very simply put, you need motivation. You, as parents, need it. Your child needs it. Your whole family needs it. But *the key* to successful motivation is to know *different ways to keep going.*

Because motivation and willpower on their own won't always work. Adults and children have lives and they live them through emotions and feelings. There are going to be tough spots and down points and if you don't have the motivation to get through these moments, then you won't succeed in helping your child to lose weight and become a healthier person.

You are in control. Not only of your life, but if you are the parent, then you are responsible for your child, too. You have to be the one to take the step forward and say that you will take care of yourself and your family. And that everyone in your family is going to have to work together towards the same goal, because even if there is just one person not on the same page, who has a different goal, or an indifferent attitude, it will have a negative effect on the whole process and wear away that motivation a whole lot quicker then it would ever do on its own. You must get everyone working together and this sounds simple enough, but it can be very difficult sometimes. So you're going to have to come up with ways in which the whole family has a goal to work to and a great reward for reaching it.

The goal for your child losing half a stone may be a trip to the ice-skating rink, but the reward for the whole family of eating healthily and doing stuff together for a month could be a day trip somewhere, like a theme park or a zoo. Something that your whole family could enjoy. Perhaps you could encourage your children to become involved in choosing where they go on holiday? The focus lies in honing in on what is of interest to each person as an individual and to the group as a whole and setting targets in relation to each.

So how do we make a start on this process? If your child is treating themselves with food (or you're helping them do it!) then try and find out why. Talk to your child and ask them how eating the food makes them feel. Is it just for that immediate gratification? That they actually felt hungry? Or that they thought it would make them feel better?

Because in the long run, food is not going to make your child feel better. Physically, or mentally. If your child is being bullied or has experienced name-calling at school, eating the food, whatever it is, healthy or not, will not improve matters. So talk to your son or daughter. Let them know that the food is not making them happy. It is contributing to their problem and making it worse. (Try to do this is an age-appropriate manner.)

Your child (and you) has got to want to change their situation. This is key. Why? Well, imagine if you got told you were about to have your wages cut in half. That I thought you could live on half the money and it would teach you to be financially clever and I thought that the extra cash you'd been getting had been making you frivolous and wasteful.

Would you like that? Of course you wouldn't. Money is important. As is food.
But, if *you* were the one to realize that you were wasting half your

salary on useless things that weren't improving your life and that you were technically chucking it down the drain and *you* decided that instead you wanted to put half of it in the bank and save up for something really great, like a holiday or a new car, then wouldn't you feel better about making the change?

You have to look at the problem and *see* what the actual problem is. If you can see the problem and where you are going wrong and take steps to change it, then you feel great. But if someone else, especially someone in authority, like a parent, suddenly decides you can't have something anymore and doesn't explain why, wouldn't you feel resentful and aim to work against them?

The child must also want to change their situation. But they have to understand what that situation is. So talk to your child and the family as a whole. Talk about food and health and problems with being overweight. Make it a game if they are very young. But always try to explain *why*, in a manner of which they'll be able to understand.

Next, be assured that *anyone* can change their bad habit. Whether it is someone who has smoked forty a day for fifty years or a heroine user. Anyone can change. The key lies in identifying the problem and then tackling it in small parts. Because as you overcome one little problem and conquer it, you're stronger to tackle the next little problem. And so on and so forth. Because little things, add up to big things.

Imagine you gave your child a target to lose a pound in weight every two weeks. In a year's time, they would have lost 26 pounds. Nearly two stones in weight. Isn't that incredible? And yet losing just one pound in two weeks seems like such a small amount. You may wonder how it could possibly be successful? But the little things add up. And also, by using that particular target, it sounds achievable to your child. One pound? They can do one pound, right? And in two weeks? Easy peasy. Your child has to think they can achieve their targets set for them. They have to know that their goals and therefore their rewards, are attainable. Otherwise, what's the point for them? If you asked your child to lose half a stone in a month they can't picture that. Six pounds? What's six pounds look like? Three bags of sugar, whoa! They're heavy! That's a lot. Suddenly they get scared. It seems difficult, they lose their confidence.

The goals and the rewards have to be attainable.

You also have to know (because this isn't just about food) what activities your child (and your family) are good at. Then encourage the child to do them. Enroll them in a club or join a league. If they don't know what they're good at, then get out there and find something they do like! By doing activities, especially out of the house, you are keeping your child activated and motivated and encouraged. They get fresh air and exercise sometimes, without even being aware that it is happening, especially if it something they enjoy. It doesn't have to be something expensive or exciting. If your child likes walking the family dog with you, then take them along. If they want to fly their kite in the local park then take them. Buy a football. They're not expensive. Or get roller skates or a skateboard. These activities don't cost huge amounts of money. Your child may even have an interest in flowers and plants, so why not get them in the garden? Teach them about growing and nurturing flowers whilst they're pulling up weeds or mowing the lawn!

There is always an activity they can do *that they will like.*

If they say they can't be bothered or there aren't any activities they like, don't believe them. They simply haven't tried. There's something out there for everyone, they've simply got to want to look! And this can be a time when those rewards we were talking about will come in useful.

Another task you ought to take care of before you start is to acknowledge and then *forget* any past failed attempts at getting your child to lose weight. Write it down. Everything. When you did it and why. How you tried to do it and your feelings about it. And then throw it away. Put the failure behind you. It's not important now. The present is important. This is important. Not what happened before. You can't move forward and help your child this time if you're stuck on focusing on the past attempt. If you expect to fail, then you will. You will sabotage your own efforts and your motivation won't even get up off the ground. Men didn't learn how to get those planes off the ground by focusing on their past failed attempts.

They looked at them. Learnt from them and then they moved on. Do the same. Don't make excuses for your past behaviour. Accept what happened, resolve to change your reaction to a similar situation and simply move on.

The next thing to do is to acknowledge that you do have the time to do this. So many healthy eating practices go out of the window after a few days or weeks because the motivation goes and suddenly a person is saying, 'I didn't have the time to make the meals/I couldn't be bothered/I was tired/I'd had a hard day' etc. Acknowledge that these times will come and resolve to react to them in a positive manner. If you've time to open your freezer, pull out a box, undo it, find a knife, pierce the clingfilm a few times and then bung it in the microwave and wait five minutes for your artificial lasagne to cook, then you've certainly got the time to go to the fridge and chop up a healthy salad and pop open some tuna instead. If your child is tired and weary or had a difficult day at school, is giving them an unhealthy calorie, fat and salt-laden food going to make them feel better? Will they feel refreshed and raring to go afterwards?

Probably not. They might want to veg out in front of the TV or computer because they continue to feel tired and, yes, why not have a few sweeties whilst the soaps are on too?

But if you persevere, and give your child something healthy and full of vitamins and nutrients, they'll feel better, more nourished, and you'll feel better for having given them something you know

62

is good for them. All the better is you get them to come out for a walk and fresh air as well! They might not feel like it, but by the time you all get back to the house you'll be glad that you did. You'll feel invigorated and more awake, less tired. And you'll also have the knowledge that you've helped your child.

Little things, remember, add up to the big things.

Be aware of using the word 'diet'. Try your best not to say it. Even to a child, it has negative implications. It has a stereotyped image of people going hungry and craving chocolate and doughnuts whilst dining on a celery stick and lettuce leaf. People think they won't have enough food and spend most of their day feeling hungry, clutching their stomachs to prevent the pangs of hunger and rumbling of their tummy. And diets don't usually work anyway. They can be restrictive and may seem successful whilst you're on them, but the second you come off, the weight can pile right back on again and yo-yo dieting is bad for the health.

We're not going to be putting your child, or your family, on a diet. We're just going to re-educate the way you think and deal with food and activity. What you buy, what you cook, what you give as snacks, how you keep yourself occupied during your spare time. It's a lifestyle change. Not an exercise and dieting program.

Don't expect this to happen overnight either. It's not realistic. This is a process that will take months. You're going for a goal that is long-term. Acknowledge that. Accept it. Otherwise you'll be right back on the sugary stuff within the week. So knowing that this is a long-term goal, try and think through your family's day, and especially your child's day, from the second they get up, to the time they go to bed.

What are their snack times? When do they reach for the biscuits? Where are the times where they might sag in front of the television. Because these are the moments you need to be prepared for. Accept that they'll come, accept that sometimes, your child will feel the need to just reach for something out of the cupboards to put in their mouths.

This is mostly habit.

Not because they're hungry. And anyway, soon you'll be providing them with delicious, healthy meals and they won't want to snack as often. And if they do get the nibbles in between meals for whatever reason, you'll be prepared with some tasty alternatives for them to try that won't help clog their arteries or contribute to future diabetes.

Work with your child through this process. Give them some other thoughts to help them change their outlook. Don't let them think that "You're horrible! Jimmy's Mum lets him have chocolate when he wants!" Make it into a great treat. Sound enthusiastic. Say, "We don't need chocolate all the time, because we've got fruit lollies!" (Made with fresh fruits, ice and set in the freezer at home).

One important thing to remember when you are discussing this new initiative with your child. *Never make negative_comments about their weight.* By negative, I mean along the lines of "You don't want to be a fat pig all the time, do you?" or "You wobble more than jelly does. So something had to be done!"

That's not the way to get a child to cooperate, no matter how sweetly you say it or whether you have a smile on your face and you know you're only joking. Children don't get sarcasm. (Teenagers, maybe)

So let them learn from example. Be their role model. Show them how enthusiastic you are about trying new foods, eating fruit and vegetables and remarking on the wonderful tastes of all this new food they are going to start eating. Let them see that Mum and Dad are quite happy to walk to the paper shop and play in the back garden with them. That swimming can be fun or even just dancing to some music at home.

And one biggie. This is key.

Clear your kitchen of junk food. Get rid of it. If you don't want to waste money by throwing it away, then store it somewhere safe where it can't be got at and if everyone sticks to the new program, then they can pick one item from the bag once a week. But you must remove the temptation. If the child can see it, they'll want it. Instead, make sure there is always a bowl of fruit out on the table. It's not expensive. You can get plenty of fruit for the same amount of money you'd spend on biscuits, cakes, chocolates, sweets and ready meals or take outs.

Your child cannot eat what isn't there.

Don't focus or worry about the fact that you might upset them. That your child may 'hate you' for a while. They'll get over it. Your child does not always have to like you. (They never do anyway!) Just remember the final goal in all of this. You are saving your child from a future of ill health and premature death.

Food is not a reward. It's functional.

We'll find other treats for them.

The Self

Self-esteem can be a huge issue and if your child is experiencing huge problems at school because of name-calling or bullying because they are overweight, then you need to speak to your school and even, maybe, ask if your child can speak to someone about how they feel.

Being bullied for being overweight can be a vicious circle. A child gets hurt by the experience and comes home and tries to make themselves feel better by eating a packet of sweets or crisps. They might enjoy the immediate reward of the taste and the feeling in their stomach, but in the long run, it just adds to the problem. The food is not their friend. It isn't making them feel better.

The child just thinks it is.

But there is one last thing I want to tackle about some children being overweight and it can be emotive and you might not want to consider it, but it does happen. So I need to mention it.

Some children will make themselves overweight to deliberately become unattractive to prevent unwanted advances. Child abuse. Yes. It is a sad fact of today's society and I don't like to think of it happening, but it does.

Out of the thousands of parents that might pick up this book, one or two might have a child that fits into this category. In this case, you need to know about it. It needs to be reported and help found for the child. Because until that huge problem is sorted and *stopped*, the weight issue, is the least of your problems.

5

HEALTHY FOOD AND HEALTHY LIFE!

Unless you've been living in a cave, I think it's quite safe to say that most people know what is healthy food and what's not. But if there are any doubters out there, I'll list a *few* of the bad foods to avoid and *some* of the good, healthy food, we all ought to be eating.

Bad Foods
- Sweets
- Chocolate
- Biscuits
- Cakes
- Some ready-meals
- Some take-away foods
- Heavily salted crisps
- Fried food dripping in fat
- Food encased in batter
- Ice-creams
- Desserts
- Fizzy drinks

Now before I get lynched, let me just plainly state that I have listed these foods because they are unhealthy if you eat them all the time to the exclusion of healthy foods and you are putting on weight because of your intake of these foodstuffs. In moderation, and as a treat, I have no problem with anyone having any of these items. (But it must be a treat/small portion/one a week kind of thing!)

<u>Good Food</u>
- Fresh fruit
- Fresh vegetables
- Lean meats
- Unbattered fish

And there's nothing to say that none of these good foods can't be jazzed up with some herbs and spices (which are calorie free!) Eating unprocessed foods does not have to be boring. There are plenty of fresh sauces to make from simple, uncomplicated ingredients.

And I also know you don't want to be stuck in the kitchen every day for hours preparing food, so it's probably best to make big batches of everything and freeze it in individual portion sizes. This will free up your time as a family to go out and be active!

What your child (and family) eats will affect them not only now, but in the long term too. You've got to aim for a *balanced* diet, because they *are* growing and need all the nutrients and bone building food. A balanced diet will also assist their body's ability to fight off infections, stay healthy, have energy, aid concentration and stay positive.

But what is a 'balanced diet'? Simply, it's a wide variety of food that contains all the vitamins and essentials that a body needs to stay healthy and fit. There should be at least five portions of fruit and vegetables every day. There should be carbohydrate-based foods (such as bread, rice, pasta, potatoes), calcium rich foods (dairy products, tinned fish), healthy fats (such as from nuts, oily fish) and protein foods (lean meat, fish, eggs, pulses).

Doesn't sound too bad, does it? And if your child is vegetarian, they could have an extra amount of dairy (protein rich) food instead of meat, or they could have extra pulses/lentils, etc. Don't serve the food on huge plates. Because then you'll be tempted to 'fill' the plate to make it look like they're getting a good portion. Use smaller plates and don't pile it high. They don't need a mountain of food if they're eating a balanced diet.

When you prepare the food for your whole family, remember not to add salt. Yes it adds flavour, but we all eat too much salt and we need to reduce that. If you do still want to add it during your cooking, then make sure your child does not also add it to their plate when the food is served. Use less than you normally would.

If your child wants a drink with their meal, then give them water or milk. It won't harm their teeth or add to their calorie count the way fizzy pop or squash might.

So how do you get your kids to eat fruit and veg?
The obvious way would be to always make sure there's a bowl of

fruit available for snacks. Eating five a day can contribute towards preventing heart disease and cancers in later life, so it's very important indeed. You could try and make it a game if they're very young. Make a chart with the colours of the rainbow and see if they can eat as many 'colours' each day as they can. Older children may require different tactics. Chips don't count as a portion. Neither do potatoes in any form, I'm afraid!

Try adding some fruit to breakfast cereal. Sprinkle some raisins or chopped banana on top. Put fruit in their lunchboxes for school. Make your own pizza and top it with lots of vegetables like red peppers, mushroom, onion and tomatoes and then cover them with cheese. You could even make the base of the pizza from sweet potato if you wanted to try something a little different!

Make your own soups and add lots of vegetables before blitzing it with a mixer. You don't have to tell them about everything that's in it! You could also hide vegetables in a home-made curry, pie, burger or even stick them in mashed potato.

Start by asking your child what vegetables and fruits they like and make a point of including these. Then, as time passes and your child gets used to their new taste experiences, you can introduce others that they might like. Let them help you choose them. Show them around the fresh produce section in the supermarket.

At home, prepare the food together, encouraging them to taste the fruits and vegetables that can be eaten raw.

If your children get hungry between meals (and this will happen at the start when the child's body craves the high calorie sugar and salt it's always been used to) then you need to be able to provide healthy snacks for them to eat, that won't ruin their appetite for dinner and won't contribute to their weight problem. As stated before, make sure there is no junk food in the house. If its not there, the child can't eat it. Provide fruit, or offer them a slice of toast with Marmite on. Or you could tempt them with a chunk of cheese, nuts, a low-fat yoghurt, popcorn, rice cake or sticks of celery or carrot with a chickpea dip. (Obviously not all at once!)

Take your child's mind off their hunger (or boredom) by asking them to help you prepare the meal and serve it. They could lay the table and get out the cutlery. Praise them for doing so. Let them know that if they help you each day in the kitchen then at the end of the week they can have a treat, like a family trip to the local swimming pool. Something that involves activity. Not chocolate! And I'm hoping this is obvious, but I'll reiterate it anyway, but when you serve up your new healthier meals, serve them to the whole family. Not just the child or children that you wish to lose weight. This is about the family *as a whole.*

Now I know that some children can be picky about what they eat and you may even now be thinking 'it's all very well you telling me to get my child to eat better, but you don't know my Susan!' etc, etc. No. I don't know your particular child. How could I? But I do know that no child will volunteer to stay hungry for ever. They may be using mealtimes as a great opportunity to wind you up. Knowing that you get mad and will put on a fantastic display of parental frustration. When a child realizes that they have control of what goes in their mouths, then they tend to exercise that right. All of them. At some point.

Just ignore it.

That's right. As simple as that. If they get no reaction whatsoever, then they soon tire of the game and realize there's no point to it. Why be hungry intentionally if Mum and Dad aren't going to put on a show? They figure they might as well eat something. Continue to eat your own food and chat happily to those at the table that are eating. When your picky eater realizes that instead of being the centre of attention, they're actually being ignored instead, they'll soon want to be a part of the happy family dynamic and will start to eat. As soon as your child starts eating their vegetables then turn to them, smile and include them in conversation.

You'll get a much happier child out of it and mealtimes will no longer be the battleground they have always been. (I've tested this theory and it *does* work. I have four children, whose only focus was to get to pudding as quickly as possible. But to do that, they had to have empty plates and pudding consisted of yoghurts or fruit attractively displayed on a plate.)

But to eat all this healthy food, a child needs a healthy appetite. Fresh air and activity is all they need and you don't have to spend money on expensive activities. Walking, running, dancing. These all help. You could fly a kite in a park, or go roller-skating or bike-riding. A ball game in the back garden? I've always enjoyed setting up an impromptu game of musical chairs just for the heck of it. I let the music play for quite a while so by the end of the game, they've done a fair bit of running around. The key is to get your child active without making them realize they're doing so.

Tell a child they've got to exercise and you get a huge sigh of boredom or disgust. Ask them if they want to help you wash the car and they can be in charge of the spray gun and they'll have their coat and wellies on before you can say 'water fight'. All it needs from you is consistency and effort.

Your child will quite quickly fall into these new habits when they realize the old calorie-laden foods are no longer forthcoming and you expect them to help you out. And you know what else? By encouraging your child in activities as a family group, you'll be giving them the greatest gift, apart from their health. You'll be giving them the gift of *you*.

What child doesn't want to spend more time with Mum or Dad? They want to have fun with you, they want your approval, they want you to see what they can do. The more you take the opportunity to go out there and have fun with them, the more they'll ask to do it with them. And what better gift for you, too?

6

INVOLVING THE CHILD IN CHOICE.

Hopefully, you'll have noticed, especially in the last chapter, that I mentioned involving your child in the choice of foods or activities. The importance of their involvement is not to be overlooked. Because if they feel that they are helping you, that they are involved in a change, rather than just having it forced upon them, they will be much more cooperative than you could ever have dreamed of them being.

Imagine you want to move house. You need somewhere bigger/smaller for whatever reason. You come home one day and tell your child you've found a place and that you're all going to be moving in three months time. Get packing. What do you see? Shock on their faces? Fear? Anxiety? Anger, maybe?

Then imagine, you discuss with the family as a whole, that you need to move house. You'd like the children to come around and view houses with you. That they can have a say on what they think to individual properties. That they can see if the bedrooms are going to be big enough for them or whether they like the look of the area.

Now what do you see? Excitement? Happy faces?

Okay, it might be a bit extreme using something as big as moving house as my point of demonstration, but surely you could imagine the differences? Apply the two scenarios to anything. Moving school, perhaps? In any scenario you come up with, I can promise you that if you involve your child in the choice of something new, it encourages them and makes them less scared. They feel in control and that there opinions are worth hearing. That they are valued.

You don't have to be moving house. This involvement takes shape in many forms.

First of all, in the dejunking of the kitchen! Get your child to grab the bin liner and hold it whilst you systematically work your way through the cupboards getting rid of the crisps and biscuits. Yes, they may get upset at the apparent loss of all their 'goodies' but explain to them that they're not disappearing forever. That if they're good, they can have a choice of one of the items from the bag once or twice a week. But if you decide they can have something once a week, then stick to it! And make it the same day. Otherwise, they'll soon work out that they can confuse you and make you think that they haven't had anything yet that week and that you promised and 'oh, Mum, it's not fair!'

Stick to your rules and rewards. Stray off the path and you're a gonner!

Now…once you've cleared your kitchen, you might be in for a shock. Are your cupboards practically bare? Had you not realized just how much junk food you purchased?

In which case, you need to go shopping and replenish the bare shelves.

Why not see if your child can help you write a shopping list of all the new foods they're going to be helping you to choose?

Then take your child with you. Go straight to the fresh produce, which in most cases is right at the entry to most supermarkets. Get a selection of fruits and vegetables that you know your child likes and one or two others to try. Make sure you buy enough for two or three day's worth of meals. This way the nutrients won't deplete, you'll always have fresh and you won't have to go every day with a screaming child that gets bored quickly.

Remember that you're in charge of what goes in the trolley! The child may ask, but if its laden with salt or sugar then say 'no. We don't buy that anymore'. Don't say anything else. Don't allow yourself to get embroiled in a verbal argument or bargaining. They'll soon get the picture when Mum or Dad don't say anything else. You can't have an argument on your own. They may become sullen and troublesome, but try to distract them. Encourage them to read what's next on the list and ask them if they can spot it before you. Make it into a game.

Avoid the aisles with sweets and biscuits!

Just go past them. don't mention them or draw attention to them. If your child pulls at the trolley to go down one of them just take the child's hand and say again, 'no. We don't buy that anymore.'

Of course you can't buy everything that is fresh. You'll need a few canned products or something out of a packet to start. If you do, then check the labeling. Make sure it doesn't have added colors, flavorings, sweeteners or preservatives.

Check that the salt content is not high and that it isn't laden with calories. If this seems boring or time-consuming, recognize that you'll only have to do it a couple of times before you know and that you could involve your child by helping you to read the main label, whilst you read the ingredients and nutrition labeling.

Don't shop if you're hungry. You'll all be tempted into throwing something into the trolley as 'one last treat'. Think about it. You'll be sabotaging your efforts before you've even started and what's the point of that? You're also meant to be leading by example and showing your child that you are a strong individual. Why would they stick to something if you don't?

At the till, ignore any pleas for the sweets on display. Many shops have now prevented this, but there are still one or two that continue to use 'pester power' to up their profits and takings. Remember, they're only in the business to keep your custom and make money. They aren't there to monitor your child's health or calorie intake.

You are.

But shopping and kitchen dejunking are not the only ways to involve your child.

Does your child have a lunchbox at school? It would be so easy to just stick sandwiches, a packet of crisps and a juice in it each day. Every parent knows the struggle to create a healthy lunchbox to fit in with school guidelines and know that their child won't get hungry.

But remember what we said before?

Your child can only eat what is there. If all you provide them with each day are healthy lunches in their box for school, then they won't starve themselves. They'll begin eating it all to prevent sitting in the classroom mid-afternoon with hunger pangs in their belly knowing its an hour until home time.

So what to provide in a lunchbox? Every day? That's varied and interesting and doesn't contravene school rules? Well, a drink, obviously. This could be milk or water. Or you could dilute some fresh fruit juice with water and keep it in a small flask. Alternatively, you could put fresh fruit juice in a flask with ice cubes. By lunchtime, they'll have melted and mixed.

A portion of fruit and/or a portion of vegetable sticks. Carrot and cucumber are good as well as being tasty they're very refreshing and naturally sweet.

If you provide sandwiches, make sure they're healthy, not filled with jam. Try an egg salad sandwich or a cheese salad sandwich. You could add a little home-made coleslaw to them too for extra flavor.

What about a low-fat yoghurt? Or a plain one for your child to add their piece of fruit to?

Most schools prefer you not to send your child to school with nuts in their lunchboxes because of possible peanut allergy, so try and avoid these here, but provide them at home. You could vary your sandwich fillings or not use bread at all some days and wrap the salad up in strips of ham or chicken. You could include home made pizza strips or a boiled egg.

There are many different variations for your child and all of them will fill them up for the day and provide enough energy for school and home.

Ask your child to choose what goes in their lunchbox. 'Do you want vegetable sticks today? Or coleslaw?'
'Could you help me slice the cucumber?'
'Would you like to pick which yoghurt goes in today?'
And why not give them a surprise in their lunchbox? Instead of a

packet of chocolate buttons, why not include a funny drawing? They'll open their lunchboxes with great anticipation each day. Mealtime will become fun as they try to guess what Mum or dad has put inside of it today. Kids love finding short little notes from Mum or Dad in their lunchboxes.

And what about snacks for the school day?

Some schools have tuck shops and a lot of these will sell fruit or small cartons of milk, but what if they don't? You'll want to ensure that your child is having a great, healthy snack at school and make them feel like they're not missing out, especially when all their friends are tucking into chocolate bars. So if the tuck shop does not sell fruit or anything healthy, do two things.

Firstly, do not allow your child to go into school with money. This can be easier said than done, but if they don't have the money to purchase rubbish, then they won't be eating it either. Explain your reasons why you do not wish for them to be taking in money, but also talk to the school and see if they can alter what they sell in their tuck shop.

Secondly, make your own healthy snacks at home for your child to take in. These snacks can be any of the foods we've already mentioned. A small tub of pre-washed grapes, an apple, etc. But there are some great snacks you can make in batches each weekend to get your child through all those tempting, hungry break times.

Below are four recipes for healthy snacks that have been reproduced with permission from a book called <u>Healthy Eating For Kids</u> (Anita Bean, A&C Black, 2004, ISBN 0713669179). It contains many food ideas for main meals too and is worth a look if you want to continue to make and prepare all of your children's food.

All of these recipes are easy to do and require no special cookery skills.

<u>Fruit Muffins</u>
(Made with wholemeal flour, these are rich in fibre, iron, B vitamins and antioxidants. This recipe makes 12 muffins.)
- 125g (4oz) white self-raising flour
- 125g (4oz) wholemeal self-raising flour
- Pinch of salt
- 40g (1½ oz) soft brown sugar
- 2tbsp (30ml) rapeseed oil
- 1 size 3 egg
- 200ml (7fl oz) milk
- 85g (3oz) raisins or sultanas

1. Pre-heat the oven to 220°C/425°F/Gas mark 7.
2. Mix the flours and salt together in a bowl.
3. Add the sugar, oil, egg and milk. Mix well.
4. Stir in the dried fruit.
5. Spoon into non-stick muffin tins and bake for 15-20 minutes until golden brown.

Gingerbread People

This recipe is low in fat and makes about 10 gingerbread people.

* 60g (2oz) butter or margarine
* 125g (4oz) soft, dark brown sugar
* 4tbsp (60ml) golden syrup
* 225g (8oz) plain flour
* ½ tsp (2.5ml) bicarbonate of soda
* 2tsp (10ml) ground ginger
* ½tsp (2.5ml) cinnamon
* 1 egg

1. Pre-heat the oven to 190°C/375°F/Gas mark 5.
2. Grease a baking sheet.
3. Melt the butter or margerine, sugar and syrup in a saucepan.
4. Add the remaining ingredients and combine quickly to form a soft dough. If it is too sticky, add a little extra flour.
5. Roll the dough out on a floured surface then use a cutter to make the gingerbread people (or whatever shape you wish!)
6. Place the cut out shapes on the baking sheet and bake for 10 minutes or until firm to the touch and golden brown.
7. Place on a wire rack to cool. You can decorate with a little icing, if you wish and add raisins or sultanas for features.

Wholemeal Raisin Biscuits

These biscuits are far healthier than shop-bought ones, lower in sugar and higher in fibre. This recipe makes about 20 biscuits.

* 225g (8oz) wholemeal plain flour

- 40g (1½oz) brown sugar
- 85g (3oz) raisins
- 2tbsp (30ml) rapeseed oil
- 1 size 3 egg
- 4tbsp (60ml) milk

1. Pre-heat the oven to 180°C/350°F/Gas mark 4.
2. Mix the flour, sugar and raisins together in a bowl.
3. Stir in the oil, egg and milk and lightly mix together until you have a stiff dough.
4. Place spoonfuls of the mixture onto a lightly oiled baking tray.
5. Bake for 12-15 minutes until golden brown.

Cereal Bars

These highly nutritious bars are made from oats and muesli which provide slow-release energy. They are lower in fat than commercial cereal bars and also full of fibre. This recipe makes about 12 bars.
- 175g (6oz) oats
- 85g (3oz) no added sugar muesli
- 150g (5oz) dried fruit mixture
- 3tbsp (45ml) honey (clear or set)
- 2 egg whites
- 175ml (6 fl oz) apple juice

1. Pre-heat the oven to 180°C/350°F/Gas mark 4.
2. Mix the oats, muesli and dried fruit in a bowl.
3. Warm the honey in a small saucepan until it is runny.

4. Add to the bowl.

5. Stir in the remaining ingredients.

6. Press the mixture into a lightly oiled 18x28cm (7 x 11in) baking tin.

7. Bake for 20-25 minutes until golden.

8. When cool, cut into bars.

As you can see, these recipes are simple and use good quality ingredients. And the best thing about these recipes (as with most recipes) is that you can use your imagination with the ingredients!

Just don't make them alone! Get your child involved. Ask them how they could experiment with flavours. Could they perhaps stew some apple and add it to the cereal bars too?

It's simply a case of feeling confident with what you are doing, but if you can get your child to help you shop for ingredients, as well as make the snacks and prepare their own foods, then they'll be more interested in it, and more likely to eat it.

Remember! They are *not* on a diet. No food is banned. Not really. They can still have foods that are being 'withheld' as their weekly reward. And if you set a good example as a whole family, then the child will cooperate to fit in with everyone else.

With activity, involve your child too with finding ways of becoming more active.

Can they walk to school? Cycle? Skate? Get them to create a 'school-run bingo'. You create a list of things they each have to see on the way to school (for example, a post box, a spiky leaf, a blue car). It can be anything and everything. This then keeps their mind busy as they walk without them realising they are being active!

Take them swimming during the week. Don't just leave it for weekends. And get in the pool yourself. See if the leisure centre runs any fun aqua classes for children and try and book them a place. Kids love splashing about and it might be preferable to the idea of swimming back and forth doing lengths or widths.

Also, you don't have to ban the television altogether. Even though too many children vegetate in front of the 'goggle box' you can also ask your child to help choose their 'TV Time'. Allocate them one hour of television a day. They get to choose that hour as long as they have completed any homework first. But when that hour is over, turn off the set and get them up and about, whether its's an impromptu dance, game of charades or a kickabout in the back garden. (If your child has a TV set in their room, discuss with your partner and child/the family as a whole, its removal!)

Or, you can set the rule that they can have an hour's worth of telly *only when* they have had an hour's worth of activity FIRST. (This is preferable.) Turn off any televisions whilst meals are being eaten and make sure everyone sits at the table for quality family time. Do not allow anyone to eat from a tray in another room.

If they do this for a week, celebrate by having a fish and chip supper! Only instead of frying the chips, cut your own potatoes and toss them in a little olive oil, sprinkle with paprika for flavour and bake in the oven. Buy some cod pieces and coat in flour, then beaten egg and then wholemeal breadcrumbs before baking for some crunchy, tasty, *healthy* fish. Get the kids involved by getting them to do the gooey bits! They'll love using their hands to toss the potatoes in oil and spice and then dipping and coating the fish. Just ensure that the portions are sensible. Don't go overboard and don't allow copious slices of bread and butter or added salt and vinegar. Get them to squeeze some lemon juice over the fish instead, it tastes great.

So what about menu ideas, I hear you ask?

Personally, I'm averse to saying that someone must follow a specific weekly diet whereas on Day One they all eat a certain type of breakfast, lunch and dinner with an allowed list of snacks and so on and so forth on Day two, three, four, etc, etc.

Meals should be fun and enjoyable. If you feel like you're following a set of rules (especially children) then you tend to want to rebel, as I'm sure you'll experience when you take away all those bad snacks from your kitchen!

So what I'm choosing to do instead, is to provide you with a list of different, healthy ideas for breakfasts, lunches and dinners. You don't have to eat these foods all the time to a rigid structure.

They're just suggestions. And hopefully, because you're all feeling motivated by what magnificent changes you are all going to make to your health as a family group, you'll want to try them.

I've tried not to list expensive foods, or hard to find products. I've also tried to keep the meals simple as not everyone has the time or skill to create culinary masterpieces.

Please remember that these ideas are mainly aimed at the child that you are encouraging to eat healthily, but are also going to be eaten by the whole family. When arranging the food on the plate, try not to just lay it out as you might normally do. Try and make it look attractive. Or, ask your child to help you serve the food, involving them with how it is laid out and served as this will also encourage them the more to eat what they have helped to prepare.

7

MEAL SUGGESTIONS
BREAKFAST IDEAS

- Sugar-free muesli with milk (semi-skimmed)
- Cereal (served with chopped fresh fruit)
- Cereal (topped with natural yoghurt)
- Two slices of wholemeal toast (topped with peanut butter or fat free spread)
- Two slices of wholemeal toast with grilled tomatoes
- Porridge (no sugar added)
- Fruit smoothie
- Boiled or scrambled egg on wholemeal toast
- Fresh fruit

MIDDAY LUNCH
- A healthy lunchbox if at school.
- Wholemeal sandwich filled with salad and a banana.
- Wholmeal sandwich filled with tuna, healthy mayo and sweetcorn. Yoghurt.
- Wholemeal sandwich filled with salad and cheese. Box of raisins.
- Wholemeal sandwich filled with egg salad. Dried apricots.
- Wholemeal pitta bread filled with any of the above.

- Home-made pizza topped with fresh vegetables and grated cheese.
- Jacket potato with grilled bacon or baked beans.
- Jacket potato with mixed salad.
- Vegetable crudites, breadsticks and hummus dip.
- Grilled or poached chicken breast and salad.
- Grilled or poached fish with salad.
- Pasta with home-made tomato sauce and salad.
- Home-made soup and a bread roll

EVENING DINNER

- Pasta, grilled or poached chicken and green salad.
- Home-made spaghetti bolognese
- Rice, grilled or poached chicken and tomato salsa
- Home-made vegetable curry and rice
- Jacket potato, grilled mushroom, tomato and bacon
- Steamed or poached fish with ratatouille
- Toad-in-the-hole with a selection of vegetables
- Home-made lasagne
- Home-made burgers and oven potato wedges (sprinkled with paprika)
- Tuna and pasta bake, green salad.
- Fish pie with a selection of vegetables
- Home-made fishcakes and jacket potato topped with sweetcorn
- Low-fat tacos, filled with lean mince, peppers, onion and mushroom

- Roast chicken with vegetables and roast potatoes
- Mashed potato, grilled sausages and peas

SNACKS

- Fresh fruit
- Natural yoghurt
- Crackers and cheese
- Nuts
- Vegetable crudites
- Raisins and sultanas
- Breadsticks
- Wholemeal toast with yeast extract
- Small fruit smoothie

As I'm sure you can see from the above, this is just a small selection of cheap, easy, yet *healthy* ideas you can have for meals as a family. Always serve water with meals, or milk, and be sensible with portion sizes.

Regarding some of the menu ideas, you may worry about how to do a lasagne, say. Or not know how to cook spaghetti bolognese from scratch. If so, either follow the general recipe ideas below, or go to your library and peruse their food and cooking section. The vast range of cookbooks these days offer plenty of different ideas and if you remember that none of these recipes are cast in stone, you can have fun with your child adding your own extra special ingredients to give your meals a personal touch!

For spaghetti bolognese:

When making spaghetti bolognese, you really do want to use a good quality mince, so why not use a chicken or turkey mince? This dish does not always have to be beef or lamb. Start by heating some olive oil in a pan or wok and saute the mince until it is cooked properly and has started to brown off. Add any onion and garlic and fry until it has softened. Add any vegetables of choice (I use tomatoes, celery, mushroom, kidney beans) and cook until they feel tender. Meanwhile, boil a pan of water and add the spaghetti. It should take between ten and twelve minutes to cook nicely. To the mince, add either a small tin of chopped tomatoes or use a spaghetti bolognese mix and add according to the packet. Drain the pasta and arrange on the plate, serving the bolognese on top.

For a home-made pizza base:

There are two varieties of pizza base you can make and both are equally tasty to use (and the second one means you can sneak in that extra vegetable!)

For the first one, mix eight ounces of self-raising flour with a teaspoon of baking powder and a tiny pinch of salt in a bowl. Rub in forty grams of unsalted butter or margerine using your fingers until the mix resembles breadcrumbs. Add 150ml of semi-skimmed milk with a fork until the mix comes together to form a rough dough. Roll or press the dough into a large circle, or separate to make smaller pizzas and place them on a baking tray. The base is ready for toppings of your choice, but I suggest plenty of vegetables, sweet red peppers especially. But you could also add cooked cubed chicken, cooked pieces of grilled bacon or even cooked mince and chillies!

For the second variety of pizza base, it really couldn't be simpler and I have to add my husband and children are particularly fond of this one! Peel and cube some sweet potatoes and boil in a pan of unsalted water. (You don't just have to use sweet potatoes, you could use a mix of white and sweet, if you wished.) When soft, drain and mash well. Use the mash to spread out into a circular pizza shape and it is ready for topping!

<u>For home-made burgers:</u>
You'll need to saute (in olive oil) your onion first for about five minutes or until soft. Remember to have chopped these quite small first. Then with your meat, whether it's beef, turkey or chicken, you'll need to mince or chop it finely and in a bowl, mix it with your sauteed onions, wholemeal breadcrumbs and any seasoning you wish to add (though avoid salt. Get the kids to do this by hand! They'll love it. Just make sure they wash their hands first and then afterwards.) Add some black pepper if required and add an egg yolk for binding. Then form your burgers into however many you need, dust them with flour and then fry in olive oil over a medium heat until they're golden brown and cooked all the way through. (A good way of getting extra goodness into your child, is to add garlic to the first stage. They won't even notice!)

For a curry:

This recipe is fabulous for varying your ingredients and is an excellent one for personalising. Start by heating some olive oil in a pan and then add your meat of choice, chicken and turkey are both very good, but make sure they are cut into strips. Cook until done. Put them to one side on some kitchen towel whilst you wait. To the pan, add some chopped onion and garlic and saute until soft. Add a couple of tablespoons worth of curry paste (there are a variety in the shops so make sure you choose a healthy option), a tin of chopped tomatoes (or fresh if you prefer) and any vegetables that you wish (I tend to add mushroom, peas, carrot and cauliflour) and heat through until the sauce begins to bubble. Simmer for about ten to twelve minutes, stirring occasionally. Next, return the chicken to the pan and stir in with a handful of sultanas or tinned chickpeas and cook for another ten to fifteen minutes. Serve with rice and/or salad.

For fish pie:

Boil your potatoes in unsalted water for about fifteen minutes before draining and mashing them, mixed with a little milk. In the oven, submerge your cod and/or haddock pieces in a dish of milk. Cook for about six minutes and then remove the fish, saving the milk for the sauce. Break your fish into small pieces. In another pan, melt a little unsalted butter, add some leeks or vegetable of choice and cook until soft. Stir in a tablespoon or two of plain flour and add the milk that was used earlier, stirring all the time, otherwise you may get lumps. Continue to do this until the sauce mixture has thickened. You may season this with a little salt and black pepper. Combine all the ingredients together and place in a baking dish suitable for the oven. Cover the fish with the mashed potato and sprinkle some grated cheese on the top. Use different cheese flavours until you find one you like. Then bake for about twenty minutes until the top has turned a golden brown using a heat of 190°C/Gas mark 5.

For home-made fish-cakes:

This recipe really is the most versatile one of the lot and can include many different tastes and varieties. Plus it has the added advantage of you being able to really involve your child in the preperation process. Cook your potatoes in boiling unsalted water until soft and drain. At the same time, poach your fish of choice (use a variety if you can. Don't feel you have to stick with salmon and cod) for about ten minutes in the oven and drain off the water. Flake your fish, checking for any bones if your fishmonger has not previously prepped the fillets. Mash the potato using milk and unsalted butter and add a sprig or two of parsley for flavour. Mix in the fish by hand and then shape into how many fishcakes you require. Shallow fry the fishcakes in olive oil until they are cooked through and nicely browned and drain on kitchen paper before serving with some nice potato wedges cooked in the oven or a green salad.

For Toad-In-the-Hole:

Use four ounces of plain flour, one egg and half a pint of milk and mix well. Select a quality sausage and grill under a medium heat for about ten minutes. When cooked, transfer to a baking dish and pour the batter over. Bake in the oven at about 190°C/Gas mark 5 until the batter has risen and has crisped nicely to your requirements. Serve with a selection of fresh seasonal vegetables.

For Tuna Pasta Bake:

Cook your pasta shapes and drain off. In another pan, using olive oil, saute some onions and garlic until they have softened. (You can also add leeks, celery, etc.) To make a sauce, melt a tablespoon of unsalted butter and add a tablespoon of cornflour and then half a pint of semi-skimmed milk, stirring continuously to prevent lumps. Wait for sauce to thicken. In a baking dish, layer vegetables of your choice (I use a variety of peas, mushroom, leek and celery) then add a layer of cooked pasta shapes, then a layer of flaked tuna (the healthier variety is in springwater or brine, not oil). Next add a layer of the sauce and keep repeating until your dish is full, finish off with any remaining sauce and place in the oven for about twenty minutes at 190°C/Gas mark 5.

For a home-made lasagne:

In a pan, heat some olive oil and soften up some onion and mixed peppers (red and green are best). Add your mince (ensure it is as lean as possible if you are using red meat) and cook until it has browned, then drain off the oil. To the same dish, add a tin of chopped tomatoes (get the variety with added herbs for extra flavour), some tomato puree and herbs such as thyme and basil. In the base of an oiled baking dish, set out a layer of lasagne sheets (available in any supermarket) and add a layer of the mince mix. Repeat until you end with a layer of lasagne sheets and then add some slices of cheese (again choose different varieties according to your family's tastes) and bake in the oven until the cheese has bubbled and turned a golden brown. Serve with a fresh green salad and/or jacket potato.

As you can see, a lot of these recipes are simple and easy to complete. They are not using expensive ingredients and are incredibly versatile. Use what you want to use and maybe even mix and match with another! The idea is to make food fun and interesting for your child, which is the whole point of involving them in the choice and preperation.

There are also a lot of simple puddings you could make, say, once a week and things like a sugar-free jelly with fresh fruit or a home-made rice pudding or even something as simple as stewed apple mixed with sultanas and served with some sugar-free custard, make great occasional puds. Just remember that they are not 'treats' or 'rewards'. Food should never be used for this purpose. It is quite a functional thing and is needed to fuel and feed our bodies and if eaten in the correct way, healthily and with a wide variety, then there is no reason why we shouldn't all enjoy great levels of energy and wellbeing in our day-to-day lives.

8

SUMMARY

So let's quickly recap as to what we can do to improve your child's weight issue. It may seem a lot of things to remember, but believe me, by performing certain tasks each day and making time for activity and eating well, it all becomes second nature.

Remember that you are doing this to improve your child's health, now and for the future. The health risks of being overweight or obese are many and in some cases, can be fatal. You are doing this not only for quality of life, but also life longevity.

Be motivated. Don't expect unrealistic miracles every day. Be aware that willpower will flag. You must all work together as a unit, supporting each other and helping each other when motivation flags and that desire to eat some chocolate cake becomes overwhelming! Do not use negative phrases when referring to your child or their weight. Help them build their own self-esteem, praising them with every success, even if it is as something small like choosing to eat an apple instead of asking for crisps. Keep that motivation going by only purchasing healthy foodstuffs. You cannot eat what is not there. Remove the temptation. All of it. It won't take long before you feel all the benefits of your new healthy lifestyle. Dejunk your kitchen and buy fresh products whenever you can. This is very self-explanatory, but very important. Fresh fruit and vegetables are not more expensive than what you've previously spent on ready meals or take-aways. The more fresh foods you eat, the less you'll be eating of fat-saturated, salt-laden, calorie high foods.

Do not restrict treats for your child. Just change what they are. Food is not a reward and it certainly isn't their friend. Make treats an activity based item, such as roller-skating or swimming at the local pool.

Ensure higher activity levels. Aim for at least one hour *minimum* of activity per day. This can include walking or cycling to school, their P.E. at school, dancing to some music at home or playing tag in the back yard. It doesn't have to cost money to be active and if you can be active as a family unit, then so much the better!

Involve your child in choice. This can be from shopping, to cooking, to food preperation and even serving dinner. Ask your child their opinion on these new events happening in their home. Ask them if they'd prefer carrot and cucumber sticks in their lunchbox, or celery and cheese? Make the alternative choice a healthy one too. That way, you, the adult, always wins.
Ensure the food you eat and prepare is balanced and varied. Poached or grilled chicken may be healthy, but if you eat it every single day then you're going to be missing other vital nutrients

you could be getting by eating a wide variety. Don't add salt when cooking. Use unsalted butters and don't add salt to your plate when you serve the meals. Salt is naturally present in many foods as sodium and as humans we eat far too much of it. Stop adding it.

Check food labels on those purchases that do come in a packet or tin. Choose the healthiest variety and after a while, this will become second nature. Remember, you are doing this for your child's health and wellbeing. This isn't a fad you're following. You're being responsible and giving your child the best.

Don't add sugar to breakfast cereals. Adding sugar isn't necessary if you top cereal with naturally sweet yoghurt or fresh fruit or even honey. Stop buying fizzy drinks and only give your child milk, water or diluted fruit juice. If they are old enough then they can have tea, but don't add the sugar.

Make sure they eat five portions of fruit and veg daily. This can be easily achieved by drinking fruit juice adding salad or fruit to a lunchbox and cooking vegetables at dinner and even hiding them in a sauce or soup. Make vegetables fun and see if your kids want to try and grow them outside in a pot! Involving them like this is a fantastic way for them to learn the natural process. (My eldest son took great pleasure in growing and harvesting tomatoes and runner beans, which he then prepared and ate. Normally you can't get a runner bean past his mouth!)

Have your child help you in the kitchen. They may make a bit of a mess, at first, but with practice they'll get better and isn't it nice to have a little help in the kitchen?

Start with vegetables and fruit you know your child will eat, then start adding different ones for them to try. If they don't like fruits, try mixing them into smoothies. Every child likes drinking stuff through straws! Buy curly-wurly ones or ones with their favourite character on.

Always have fruit out in a bowl. Make fruit available for snacks at any time and choose a good variety, buying fruit that is in season to maximise volume with cost.

Cut down on the time that the television is watched. Be active first as a family and when they've done that, allow them to watch the TV for about an hour a day.

Eat at the dinner table as a family and not on trays in front of the goggle box! Eating off a tray causes poor digestion and if everyone is in separate places, then what should be quality family time is lost forever.

Don't get into an argument about food. Keep it simple. Repeat that 'We don't buy that anymore' and stick to it. Ignore any tantrums and don't worry if your child shouts that they hate you. I know, it's awful to hear, but they want you to feel guilty and give in.

Imagine for a moment that you do give in. What has this achieved? You simply show your child they can get what they want by throwing a wobbly and it takes away their respect for you. You are doing this for their health. Their life. You Don't want to outlive your child. Keep that thought in mind and I bet you will stick to your guns. Tell them no and offer the fruit from the bowl.

Be realistic with portion sizes. A child does not require the same amount of food you would serve for yourself or your partner. They require less.

Remember your child won't starve if they refuse to eat what you serve. Eventually they will learn that you arent going to give in and they have got to eat what you all eat.

This eating plan is for all the family, not just your overweight/obese child. If they feel that they are being treated differently from everyone else in the family unit then you will quickly have a rebellion on your hands.

Involve your child in helping to write the shopping list, then take them with you. (My children enjoy taking it in turns to hold the calculator and add in the new price each time and seeing if it tallies with the till at the end.)

Don't shop whilst you're hungry or your child is tired. This will just result in a nightmare!

Make varied and healthy lunchboxes for meals at school. If your child has school dinners, then ask them for a menu so you know what they are eating and that way you won't replicate anything in the evening. Remember, variety and balance is key. Go to the library and get a variety of recipe books. This way you can mix and match recipes and ingredients and have fun in your kitchen.

Keep active. And that means everyone. Eating the right foods and keeping your intake balanced is only part of the solution for your child. They must be active too. They're children. They should be full of energy and want to go outside and run about. It does them no good at all to be glued to their TV sets or computer games.

In all, remember this is all for their health and wellbeing. By following this new food program and activity plan you are enriching their present life and their future.

9

USEFUL CONTACTS AND WEBSITES

This end section is a small selection of useful websites, addresses and telephone numbers that are of use to children as well as to parents. Because I do not know your child's age or height, I have not included any BMI (body mass index) charts for you to work out. This is because every child is an individual and each BMI chart on different charts seem to work on differing measurements. It's up to you to choose the correct one for you.

If you do have any concern about your child's health, you should always consult your doctor.

I wish you the very best for the future. I know you will be able to follow the ideas in this book and I'm thrilled to know that you will soon experience the joy at seeing the change in your child, and hopefully, your family.

Time together is precious and it passes quickly. Enjoy!

<u>Websites</u>

<u>www.bbc.co.uk/health/conditions/obesity2.shtml</u>

(This website is UK-based and is an excellent resource for parents.With links to the Food Standards Agency and the National Obesity Forum.)

<u>http://hcd2.bupa.co.uk/fact sheets/html/child obesity.html</u>

(This website is another excellent resource from BUPA, aimed at parents.It has printable factsheets and a link to the British Nutrition Foundation.)

<u>http://news.bbc.co.uk/1/hi/health/4756370.stm</u>

(This BBC site is a news report about the effects of obesity on children, but has some excellent links to pages about making activity fun.)

<u>http://www.health.nsw.gov.au/obesity/adult/background/backgro und.html</u>

(This is an Australian report, but is still relevant to British parents and children. It lists facts about obesity and gives hints and tips about what you can do and what to look for in selecting a healthy school. It also has a BMI calculator)

http://www.allaboutyou.com/relationships/columnists/healthykids
exerciseinschoolschriswoodhead/?dcopt=off

(This page is a good resource about how schools can help children that are at risk of being, or already are, overweight/obese.)

http://www.keepkidshealthy.com/

(This is an American site, but still excellent. It doesn't just deal with obesity, but all child-related health questions and is updated regularly.)

http://www.healthiergeneration.org/engine/renderpage.asp

(This is also an American site and has separate sections for schools, parents and teenagers.)

http://www.obesity.org/

(This is the site for the American Obesity Organisation. It has plenty of factsheets and information for parents of overweight/obese children.)

http://www.mayoclinic.com/health/childhood-obesity/FL00058

(This site supports the whole family ethos of working together to reduce obesity.)

http://www.healthinschools.org/

(This site has factsheets to download or print and a Parent's Resource Centre.)

http://www.bma.org.uk/ap.nsf/Content/childhoodobesity

(This site is from the British Medical Association and is all about preventing obesity.)

http://www.cofbc.ca/

(This is a Canadian charity focused on reducing obesity and has a forum for parents.)

http://www.parliament.uk/post/pn205.pdf

(British government policy and initiatives regarding how they will deal with the issue of child obesity.)

http://www.dh.gov.uk/PolicyAndGuidance/HealthAndSocialCare Topics/Obesity/fs/en

(The Department of Health's program for obesity targets by the year 2010.)

http://www.myhealthyworld.co.uk/wellnesseval.htm

(An interesting site that allows you to discover your 'wellness' by filling in a form about yourself. Many other links about nutrition.)

http://www.foodfit.com/

(A site filled with healthy foods and recipe ideas. US-based but still works well.)

http://www.healthrecipes.com/

(US-based.)

(This excellent UK site is filled to the brim with recipe ideas for breakfasts, lunchboxes, lunches and dinners as well as snacks and puddings that aren't filled with calories!)

http://www.vegsoc.org/

(The Vegetarian Society with information on healthy eating, aimed at parents and children.)

http://www.veganfamily.co.uk/main.html

(Vegan recipe ideas and information.)

http://www.carnegieweightmanagement.com/

(The Carnegie Weight Management program run by Leeds

111

Metropolitan University and Professor Paul Gately, a leading professor of child obesity. Here you can find out about weight camps and healthy eating as well as BMI calculators.)

http://www.kidshealth.org

(A general health website, that deals with children's health from birth to adulthood.)

http://www.food.gov.uk/healthiereating/

(A site from the Food Standards Agency giving consumer advice on healthy eating for everyone.)

http://www.eatwell.gov.uk/

(Another site from the Food Standards Agency giving practical advice for children from toddlers to teenagers.)

USEFUL READING

<u>Preventing Childhood Obesity: Health In The Balance</u>
By The Committee on Prevention of Obesity In Children, the
Institute of Medicine and Jeffrey P Koplan. Published 2005,
436pp. (National Academy Press)
ISBN-10:0309091969
ISBN-13:978-0309096961

<u>Overcoming Child Obesity</u>
By Colleen Thompson and Ellen Shanley. Published January
2006, 288pp. (Bull Publishing Company.)
ISBN-10:092352178X
ISBN-13:978-0923521783

<u>Helping Your Child Lose Weight the Healthy Way: A Family
Approach To Weight Control.</u> by Judith Levine and Linda Bine.
Published September 1996, 256pp. (Citadel Press.)
ISBN-10:1559723459
ISBN-13:978-1559723459

<u>Healthy Eating For Kids</u>
By Anita Bean. Published July 2004, 192pp. (A&C Black.)
ISBN-10:0713669179
ISBN-13:978-0713669176

Index

Emerald Publishing
www.emeraldpublishing.co.uk

106 Ladysmith Road
Brighton BN2 4EG

Other titles in the Emerald Series:

Law
Guide to Bankruptcy
Conducting Your Own Court case
Guide to Consumer law
Creating a Will
Guide to Family Law
Guide to Employment Law
Guide to European Union Law
Guide to Health and Safety Law
Guide to Criminal Law
Guide to Landlord and Tenant Law
Guide to the English Legal System
Guide to Housing Law
Guide to Marriage and Divorce
Guide to The Civil Partnerships Act
Guide to The Law of Contract
The Path to Justice
You and Your Legal Rights

Health

Guide to Combating Child Obesity
Asthma Begins at Home

Music

How to Survive and Succeed in the Music Industry

General

A Practical Guide to Obtaining probate
A Practical Guide to Residential Conveyancing
Writing The Perfect CV
Keeping Books and Accounts-A Small Business Guide
Business Start Up-A Guide for New Business
Finding Asperger Syndrome in the Family-A Book of Answers

For details of the above titles published by Emerald go to:

www.emeraldpublishing.co.uk